"What a great workout! With no pain but *a lot* of gain *The Bench Workout* tones up ALL of you in one fun conditioning program. . . . I'm impressed!"
> **—Wendy Stehling**
> bestselling author of *Thin Thighs in 30 Days*

"Nancy Burstein brings her fitness expertise to *The Bench Workout*, a great alternative to traditional aerobics that's ideal for individuals and groups alike."
> **—Russell K. Fleischmann**
> contributing editor, *Health* magazine
> program director of health and fitness,
> Bristol-Myers Squibb

"An easy-to-learn and time-efficient program, *The Bench Workout* adds a dynamic new dimension to fitness conditioning."
> **—Kathy Smith**
> star of *Kathy Smith's Weight Loss Workout* and other bestselling exercise videos

"An excellent guide to getting fit quickly and easily."
> **—Cameo Kneuer**
> Ms. National Fitness Champion
> co-author of *Cameo Fitness*

BOOKS BY NANCY BURSTEIN

30 Days to a Flatter Stomach for Women

30 Days to a Flatter Stomach for Men

The Executive Body: A Complete Guide to Fitness and Stress Management for the Working Woman

Soft Aerobics: The New Low-Impact Workout

THE Bench Workout

NANCY BURSTEIN

WARNER BOOKS

A Time Warner Company

NOTE: Before starting any new exercise program it is important that you consult your physician. This is a must if you have any serious medical conditions or if you are taking medication. Get your doctor's consent before you begin.

Warner Books, Inc., 666 Fifth Avenue, New York, NY 10103

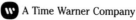 A Time Warner Company

Printed in the United States of America
First Printing: April 1991
10 9 8 7 6 5 4 3 2 1

Library of Congress Cataloging-in-Publication Data

Burstein, Nancy.
    The bench workout / Nancy Burstein.
        p.   cm.
    ISBN 0-446-39246-4
    1. Exercise.   2. Aerobic exercises.   3. Physical fitness.
I. Title.
GV481.B87   1991
613.7′1—dc20   90-48280
                                                          CIP

Book design: Giorgetta Bell McRee
Cover photo of Nancy Burstein: Don Banks
Cover design: Anne Twomey
Inside photos: Don Banks

ACKNOWLEDGMENTS

Special thanks to Anne Edelstein, Roberta Thumim, Terry Boggis, Nell Mermin, Leslie Keenan, Lisa Karl, and Don Banks.

CONTENTS

The Bench Workout

INTRODUCTION

Welcome to the Bench Workout—the dynamic fitness conditioning program designed to meet the needs of today's exercisers. A workout that involves stepping up and down on a platform while simultaneously using the upper body, the Bench Workout provides sensational cardiovascular and toning benefits, is easy to learn, requires minimal space, and adapts to all fitness levels.

While the concept of using a bench is not completely new (running stadium stairs has long been a favored training tool of athletic coaches), it has reentered the fitness field in a new format that is being touted as the "workout of the nineties." It ushers in a decade of "sensible exercise"— activity that provides health and fitness benefits without injurious biomechanical stress to the body.

Living well today means combining exercise and nutrition to create a healthy lifestyle. The Bench Workout provides an ideal exercise element (it incorporates *all* the major components of fitness) and complements a balanced diet for weight maintenance or weight loss.

By combining aerobic conditioning and strength training in one session, the Bench Workout provides a maximum return for the time you spend getting fit. While it's a low-impact activity, it can demand the energy expenditure of a high-impact run. Also in its favor, you can do the workout at home and at any time.

Whether you're looking for a new workout challenge or just beginning an exercise program, *The Bench Workout* is your guide to the very latest in fitness conditioning. It takes you through the basics: You'll learn about the right equipment, the components of a warm-up, the correct technique for bench stepping, and a variety of ways to use the bench in your workout. This book will get you started on a safe, effective, and *fun* exercise and training program.

1

WHAT YOU NEED TO KNOW ABOUT THE BENCH WORKOUT

Who'd have anticipated that the concept of stepping up and down on a bench for an aerobic, strength-building workout would sweep the country? Well, it has, and in a short time it's become the hottest trend in aerobics—and one that's here to stay. The workout has been received enthusiastically by experienced exercisers and athletes as well as by people who have shunned aerobics in the past. It's a program with great appeal for men and women of all ages and all fitness levels.

Cardiovascular conditioning is widely accepted as an essential component of a healthy lifestyle. In addition to its role in combatting heart disease, regular exercise makes people more active and vital throughout their lives and may extend longevity. Knowing this, the exerciser's quest is to select the aerobic activity that provides maximum benefits with minimum strain to the body *and is enjoyable.*

There are lots of options for aerobic exercise, but finding one that's fun and easy to learn, that will not overstress the body's musculoskeletal structure and offers an on-going challenge, can be a challenge in itself.

While traditional aerobic dance can be an effective cardiovascular conditioner, many participants find that complicated steps and routines make such a workout too difficult to master. Exercisers who run on a regular basis may suffer from injuries resulting from the impact stress of jogging. Stationary bicyclists frequently stop exercising out of boredom, and then use their expensive piece of equipment as little more than a costly clothes rack.

The Bench Workout provides the antidote to these problems. It replaces the complicated routines of aerobic dance with simple movements. We've all gone up and down stairs endless numbers of times, so the basic movement is familiar and can be accomplished even by those who never fancied themselves dancers.

Runners and high-impact aerobicizers will find that bench stepping is much gentler on the body. Studies show that the stress impact of bench stepping is similar to that experienced in walking at a pace of three miles per hour. This means there is little if any risk of injury to joints and connective tissues even though you are performing an activity that can demand as much energy as running at seven miles per hour!

The Bench Workout offers an exercise routine that is easy to learn and can be made more challenging as your fitness level increases. It's not costly, requires little space, and makes the best use of the exerciser's time by working the lower body and upper body simultaneously.

Bench stepping is an ideal aerobic/strength workout to meet the cardiovascular training requirement for a healthy lifestyle. You may choose to do the Bench Workout as your aerobic-conditioning program or include it in a cross-training regimen of several different fitness activities.

ADAPTING THE BENCH WORKOUT TO YOUR FITNESS LEVEL

The advantage of bench stepping is its flexibility in accommodating all fitness levels. You can increase the intensity level of the workout by using a higher bench and adding hand-held weights. Or, if you prefer a more moderate intensity, choose a lower bench and don't use weights. (*Newcomers to the workout should not use weights initially.*)

Bench height can range from four to twelve inches. It is recommended that newcomers to the Bench Workout start moderately with benches from four to six inches high. After your body adapts to the intensity level of this height, you can move up to a higher bench. Since it takes more effort to step up and down (working the body vertically against gravity) than to do traditional aerobics, experienced exercisers may find a lower bench is appropriate for them as well when they first begin the program.

The use of hand-held weights is optional. However, after becoming familiar with the program, intermediate- and advanced-level exercisers may opt for a more rigorous upper body workout by incorporating weights into the program. Because the arm movements are very controlled and performed to a slower tempo than traditional aerobics, the Bench Workout is an appropriate cardiovascular activity in which to use weights. Weights that range from one to three pounds can be used. However, no more than three pounds should be held in each hand even by the advanced-level bench exerciser.

Use the chart on page 6 as your guideline to bench height and weight poundage:

Level	Bench Height	Weight Held in Each Hand
Beginner	4–8 inches	None
Intermediate	8–10 inches	1–2 pounds
Advanced	10–12 inches	2–3 pounds

If you've never used the bench before, you should consider yourself a beginner, no matter what other exercises you already do. Even experienced exercisers will find that the Bench Workout makes energy demands and uses muscles differently than other workouts. Get accustomed to the program before increasing bench height and adding weights.

Generally, a beginner will need to exercise two to four times a week for about six weeks before advancing to the intermediate level. Intermediate exercisers should plan on six weeks to three months before progressing to the advanced stage.

It is important to acknowledge that your ultimate goal does not necessarily have to be a twelve-inch bench and three-pound weights. Many exercisers find they can get a good workout on a lower bench without using weights even when they've been doing the program over an extended time.

You can modify the intensity of the workout while performing the movements. If you're using weights and the workout is too demanding, simply put the hand weights down and continue the routine without them. If you're not using hand weights, discontinue the arm movements and only do the leg movements. Should the stepping actions prove too rigorous, you can stop using the bench and just perform the movements on the floor.

NOTE: While the Bench Workout can be adapted to many fitness levels and is appropriate for all ages, the program may not be suitable for some individuals. People who experience balance problems, have arthritic conditions in the knees or hips, or are extremely overweight should discuss the program with their physician before proceeding.

BENEFITS OF THE BENCH WORKOUT

How does the Bench Workout work for you? Here are the multifaceted benefits of this unique fitness program:

- *Cardiovascular conditioning.* In the fight against heart disease, the Bench Workout can help lower blood pressure, make the heart and lungs work more efficiently, and increase HDL (high-density lipoprotein) cholesterol—the good type of cholesterol.
- *Weight loss/maintenance.* As an aerobic activity, the Bench Workout is an ideal fat-burner. Fat is the body's fuel source for endurance exercise. Bench stepping's combination of low-impact movements and high energy demands (because you are moving both vertically and horizontally on the bench and using the upper body) increases the workload on the body and burns off body fat.
- *Optimum time management.* The program provides aerobic training using every major muscle group in the lower body while simultaneously conditioning the upper body.
- *Stress release.* The movements of the workout provide a gentle yet effective release of the tension that builds up in muscles during a pressured day. In addition, during exercise the body releases endorphins—natural mood elevators that alleviate depression.
- *Osteoporosis reduction.* Weight-bearing movements such as the leg movements of bench stepping can help increase bone density to counteract osteoporosis.

With all the health and time-saving advantages of the workout, you might overlook the sensational physical results supplied by the program. However, a glance in the mirror will show a well-conditioned, well-proportioned physique developing via the combination of lower-body stepping actions with upper-body conditioning.

The up-and-down stepping action of the Bench Workout

challenges every major muscle group in the lower body—
the quadriceps (front of thigh), hamstrings (back of thigh),
gluteals (buttocks), and calves. The upper body is shaped
and defined through movements that involve the deltoids
(shoulders), biceps (front of upper arm), triceps (back of
upper arm), chest, and back.

2

THE FITNESS COMPONENTS AND TRAINING GUIDELINES FOR THE BENCH WORKOUT

The Bench Workout has been designed to incorporate the primary components of a balanced fitness program:

- *Cardiovascular endurance.* The use of large muscle groups of the body creates an increased demand for oxygen over a prolonged period of time.
- *Muscular endurance.* There is an increase in the ability of a muscle to exert force repeatedly.
- *Muscular strength.* There is an increase in the maximum force a muscle can produce against resistance.
- *Flexibility.* The range of motion about a joint increases noticeably.
- *Body composition.* The relative percentage of lean body mass (bones, muscles, organs, connective tissues) versus body fat changes for the better.

To maximize the benefits of the aerobic component of the Bench Workout, you need to be familiar with the training principles for cardiovascular conditioning: overload and progression, frequency, duration, and intensity.

The overload method works like this:

To increase or improve your stamina, you increase the workload. You do this by pushing your body slightly beyond its normal capacity (this is "overload"). The workload in the Bench Workout can be varied by increasing the length of time spent exercising aerobically, increasing the height of the bench, or by using weights or adding more weight.

To prevent overexertion and possible injury, you should *progress gradually, upping only one variable at a time*. For example, a beginning exerciser on a four-inch bench might start by exercising aerobically for eight minutes, adding an extra minute or two each week, eventually building up to twenty minutes. Once the twenty-minute threshold has been reached, you have several options. You can either increase the height of the bench, add weight, or work longer. Just remember to choose only *one* variable at a time, to prevent overtaxing your body.

Overload and progression apply to three specific guidelines for aerobic exercise:

- *Frequency*: This refers to the number of times per week a person must exercise to achieve cardiorespiratory fitness. Regular aerobic conditioning will produce physiological changes such as a lowered resting heart rate and improved oxygen consumption (also known as the *training effect*). The recommended exercise prescription is a minimum of three times weekly.
- *Intensity*: During aerobic exercise the heart rate must increase to a certain level to achieve a training effect. This level of intensity is called the *target zone*.
- *Duration*: The time spent in aerobic activity can range from fifteen to sixty minutes. A minimum of fifteen minutes is required to elicit a training effect.

If you are a beginning exerciser, you may find that you are not yet adequately conditioned to perform the Bench Workout for the recommended fifteen-minute minimum. In that case you should begin exercising for a shorter time and gradually extend the length of your workout to at least fifteen minutes.

MONITORING EXERCISE INTENSITY

Monitoring how hard you are working during the aerobic component of the Bench Workout is essential for a safe and effective workout. Exercising at an intensity that is too low will not elicit the cardiorespiratory training effect, while exercising too hard can increase the potential for injury, cause overexertion, and/or make you feel overly fatigued. Your pulse will tell you if your exercise intensity is too high, too low, or at the right level.

Guidelines for achieving a training effect from aerobic exercise vary slightly, depending on which national health organization you refer to. The American College of Sports Medicine suggests an individual work out at 60 percent to 90 percent of maximum heart rate, while the American Heart Association recommends 60 percent to 75 percent. For most people, it is best not to exceed 85 percent. Beginning exercisers may feel more comfortable in the lower intensity range (60 to 75 percent—or even lower initially). Those who are more conditioned may choose to work in the higher range (75 to 85 percent).

Taking Your Heart Rate

You can easily calculate your target heart rate zone with one of the following methods.

THE MAXIMAL HEART RATE FORMULA

This formula determines your target zone based on age:

220 minus your age	=	maximum heart rate
maximum heart rate × .60	=	low end of target zone
maximum heart rate × .85	=	high end of target zone

The example for a thirty-five-year-old exerciser is:

220 − 35	=	185 (beats per minute)
185 × .60	=	111
185 × .85	=	157

The target zone for this exerciser is from 111 to 157 beats per minute.

You can either calculate your target zone with the formula given above or use the table that follows to find the heart rate zone closest to your age.

Age	Target Zone	
	60–75%	**75–85%**
20	120–150	150–170
25	117–146	146–166
30	114–142	142–162
35	111–138	138–157
40	108–135	135–153
45	105–131	131–149
50	102–127	127–145
55	99–123	123–140
60	96–120	120–136
65	93–116	116–132

Take a pulse check during your workout to determine your heart rate. Step off the bench and take your pulse by placing the tips of the index and middle fingers on the radial artery, located on the inside of the wrist in line with the thumb. A pulse can also be felt easily at the carotid artery on either side of the neck, below the jaw and to the side of the throat. Only very gentle pressure should be applied at the carotid artery, as too much pressure can cause the heart rate to slow down.

After locating your pulse, count the beats for ten seconds and multiply by six. This gives you the number of beats per minute. Be sure to keep your feet moving as you take your pulse. This will prevent blood from pooling in the legs (which can make you feel light-headed). You can just walk in place or tread your feet.

The Karvonen Formula

This method provides a more individualized heart rate: It uses the exerciser's resting heart rate, an indicator of fitness (the lower the resting heart rate, the more fit the individual), in conjunction with the heart rate based on age.

Your true resting heart rate can be calculated when you wake up in the morning. Simply sit up in bed and take your pulse for ten seconds and multiply by six. Otherwise, a modified resting heart rate can be taken prior to exercising.

The formula is as follows:

220 − your age = maximum heart rate (mhr)
mhr − resting heart rate (rhr) = heart rate reserve
heart rate reserve × intensity level + rhr = target heart rate

The example for a thirty-five-year-old exerciser with a resting heart rate of 66 who wants to work at a 60 percent level of intensity is:

220 − 35 = 185 (maximum heart rate)
185 − 66 = 119
119 × .60 + 66 = 137 (target heart rate)

At 75 percent intensity:

220 − 35 = 185
185 − 66 = 119
119 × .75 + 66 = 155 (target heart rate)

Note that heart rate and blood pressure will increase when you exercise with your arms continually at or above shoulder level, or when you grip hand weights tightly. However, the increased heart rate does not reflect an increase in your energy output. Therefore, if you exercise with raised arms or grip weights, add five to ten beats to your training zone to get an actual reflection of energy output.

Perceived Exertion

If it is difficult for you to find your pulse or if you are taking medication that affects your heart rate, perceived exertion will help you estimate how hard you're working.

On a scale of 1 to 10, ask yourself how hard you feel you are working (1 is very, very light; 10 is very, very hard). A range of 6 to 8 generally indicates the exerciser is working in the appropriate training zone. While you may be skeptical of the accuracy of this scale, studies have shown that a 6 to 8 estimate correlates with an intensity level of 60 to 80 percent of maximum heart rate when pulses are taken.

HYDRATION OR BEATING THE HEAT

The Bench Workout may cause some exercisers to perspire more heavily than usual. The energy demands of the workout increase the core temperature of the body, and perspiration is released to prevent overheating. It is essential to stay well hydrated by drinking an appropriate liquid before, during, and after the workout.

Drink one or two glasses of liquid fifteen to thirty minutes before exercising. If you are perspiring heavily during exercise, drink another glass every ten to twenty minutes to replace water losses. After the workout, drink another glass or two to rehydrate yourself.

Cold water is the best choice of fluids because it is absorbed most rapidly into the system and helps lower the body's core temperature. Beverages high in sugar (e.g., soda pop) are not recommended, as sugary drinks can cause bloating or cramping. Dilute fruit juices and sports drinks that contain sugar if you drink these during your workout.

3

GETTING THE GEAR—
YOUR BENCH, WEIGHTS,
MUSIC, AND SHOES

Equipment for the Bench Workout consists of a bench, some hand weights, and music to "step" to. The program is not costly and your investment can be kept to a minimum if you're handy with a hammer and nails and can construct your own bench. If you choose to purchase a ready-made bench, there are several available at moderate prices.

THE BENCH

Bench training has spawned a number of products designed to accommodate a variety of exercise needs. Exercisers can choose between adjustable-height and fixed-height benches. The first use support blocks to change heights in a range from four to twelve inches. Fixed-height products are available in four-, six-, eight-, ten-, or twelve-inch heights. Some benches are constructed of molded plastic, others of wood.

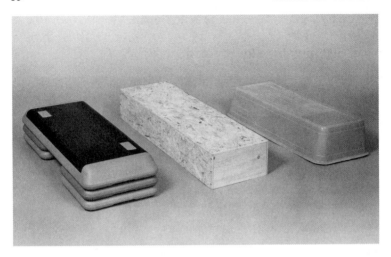

Left to right: Adjustable bench (The Step™), wood bench (Pioneer Fitness Products), molded plastic fixed-height bench (Bench-Aerobix™).

Costs range from $21 to $28 for a precut, predrilled wood bench that you assemble yourself, and from $45 to $50 for a molded plastic fixed-height bench. The adjustable-height benches (generally made of molded plastic) range in price from $60 to $105, depending upon the number of support blocks you purchase.

If you're wondering how to decide which is the best choice for you, consider your preference for increasing exercise intensity through added bench height. If you want a bench that can be adapted as your fitness level increases, opt for the adjustable-height bench, or buy two fixed-height benches of different heights (the molded plastic models can be stacked for easy storage). If you prefer a workout that is more moderate and are not interested in increasing your bench height (you can add weights or exercise longer to increase intensity if desired), then a fixed-height bench would be appropriate.

If ready-made benches are not available at your local sporting goods store, the following three manufacturers have "800" numbers for information on purchasing a bench:

Adjustable-height molded plastic benches:

The Step™
P.O. Box 6909
Marietta, GA 30065
800 833–STEP

Fixed-height wood benches:

Pioneer Fitness Products
5600 S. Quebec, Suite 218A
Englewood, CO 80111
800 822–2889

Fixed-height molded plastic benches:

BenchAerobix™, Inc.
P.O. Box 70323
Marietta, GA 30007
800 25-BENCH

If your carpentry skills inspire you to construct your own bench, you'll need some wood—maple, plywood, or pine (avoid chipcore or composition) that is ¼- to ½-inch thick—plus nails, a saw, and some nonskid paint to cover the top surface. The length of the bench should be from thirty-six to forty-eight inches, and the width should measure fourteen inches. Choose the height according to your fitness level (see page 6), and add cross supports under the surface on which you'll be stepping.

NOTE: When using a wood bench during your workout, place it on a nonskid surface such as carpeting to prevent the bench from sliding.

WEIGHTS

Hand-held weights are used in the aerobic portion of the Bench Workout. Beginners should not use any weight initially; intermediate and advanced exercisers may want the extra challenge provided by one-, two-, or three-pound weights. It is essential that the exerciser adapt to performing the workout with one-pound weights before adding more weight. Three-pound weights should be used only by advanced-level exercisers.

Small dumbbells, Heavy Hands™ (weights with handles that fit snugly in the hands), or slip-on wrist weights are good choices for the workout. All these weights should be available at most sporting goods stores.

NOTE: Under no circumstances should weights be attached to the ankles for the Bench Workout. The extra weight will overstress the lower leg, possibly leading to injury of the ankle, knee, or calf.

More weight can be used, if desired, for some of the exercises included in chapter 7, "Strengthen and Stretch on the Bench." The exercises given there are designed to build muscular strength, and since they are done in a stationary position, it is safe to increase the poundage. Exercises such as the bench press and bent-arm flyes can be done with weights of up to eight pounds for those accustomed to using weights in a conditioning program.

MUSIC

Music is an integral component of many aerobic programs, and the Bench Workout is no exception. The rhythm and dynamics of upbeat music give an energy boost and help the exerciser move at a steady, consistent pace.

The difference between music for traditional aerobics and

bench stepping is tempo. Music for this workout should be slower, to minimize the risk of injury in the stepping action. The slower pace is necessary, as it takes substantial effort to lift the body vertically and the exerciser requires a bit of extra time to place the feet carefully on and off the bench. The slow tempo also facilitates better control of upper body movements, particularly when weights are used.

Music speed is measured in beats per minute in a song. The appropriate speed for bench stepping is approximately 120 beats per minute (traditional aerobics uses speeds ranging from 130 to 160 b.p.m.). For example, the tempo of Michael Jackson's song "Billie Jean" is 120 b.p.m. Other pop selections with 120 b.p.m. include "Escapade" by Janet Jackson, "Borderline" by Madonna, and "Born in the U.S.A." by Bruce Springsteen.

Calculate the speed of your favorite music by counting the beats for ten seconds. Multiply that number by 6 and you have the beats per minute.

Should you want to use music for your warm-up, note that the tempo can be slightly faster (125 to 135 b.p.m.), since the movements are not done on the bench.

If you would prefer to purchase an audiocassette created specifically for bench stepping, one has been developed by Power Productions Inc. The 60-minute "Step Power Mix" tape includes a 10-minute warm-up, 45 minutes of bench-stepping music at 120–124 b.p.m., and a 5-minute cool-down. For more information on the tape contact:

Power Productions Inc.
P.O. Box 1200
Germantown, MD 20875
800 777–BEAT

SHOES

You must wear shoes during the workout. The shoes you select should have ample cushioning for shock absorption, enough traction to inhibit sliding on or off the bench, and lateral support for stability. An aerobic dance shoe combines these properties and is suitable for bench stepping.

4

WARMING UP
FOR WORKING OUT

The warm-up is an essential and too often neglected component of any exerciser's workout. In the haste to jump into the aerobic portion of the Bench Workout, some exercisers may be tempted to skip the warm-up and just start bench stepping. However, warming up is absolutely integral to any workout and particularly the Bench Workout. The repetitive stepping actions and upper body motions demand muscles that are limber and can move with ease.

The warm-up prepares the body for the more vigorous types of movement to be performed later in the workout. Through some easy rhythmic movements (each will help increase the body's core temperature and stimulate circulation) and static stretches (holding a position, not bouncing, to elongate muscles and connective tissues), warming up will get your body ready for bench stepping and minimize the possibility of injury. A seven- to ten-minute warm-up will:

- Increase body temperature and the amount of blood flowing to the muscles. This literally "warms" the muscles, making them pliant. Warm muscles can move more freely than "cold" muscles.
- Increase the lubricating fluid in the joints, the elasticity of

the ligaments, and the length of the tendons and muscles. This allows a fuller range of motion for the limbs.

- Raise the speed of nerve impulses, thereby helping the body to move more efficiently.
- Prepare the cardiorespiratory system so it is not suddenly overtaxed by the demands of aerobic exercise.

A good warm-up is your insurance that your body is well prepared for the Bench Workout.

THE SEVEN- TO TEN-MINUTE WARM-UP

Rhythmic Limbering

1. Briskly march in place while pumping your arms (swinging them front and back) at your sides for one minute.

2. Continue marching and use your arms in the following progression. (Repeat all arm variations 10 times.)
   a. Place hands in front of your shoulders with palms out (starting position). Stretch your arms forward and then return palms back to starting position. The arms stretch out on the first march step and back on the second.
   b. Repeat the movement, but stretch arms out to the sides at shoulder level.
   c. Repeat the movement, but reach arms to the ceiling.
   d. Repeat the movement, but press arms down toward the floor.

3. With legs about shoulder-width apart, bend your right knee back, bringing your leg slightly behind your body and your right heel up toward the right buttock. Keep your left leg slightly bent. Alternate legs. As you continue

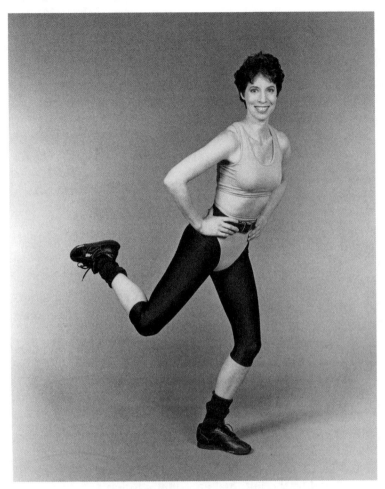

this leg movement, add the following variations for the arms. (All variations are repeated 10 times.)

a. *Bicep curl.* With arms at your sides and palms facing forward, bend the elbows and bring your palms toward the shoulders. Return arms to the starting position.

b. *Lateral arm lift.* With arms at your sides and palms facing in toward your body, lift the arms out to the side and up to shoulder height. Return to the starting position.

    c. *Triceps extension.* Bend your elbows and place your arms slightly behind your torso. The forearms should be at rib level. Extend the forearms back (straightening the arms), trying not to move your elbows. Return to the starting position.

    d. *Upper back press/chest stretch.* Lift your arms to shoulder level and bend your elbows. Gently press the elbows back as though pressing your shoulder blades together. Pull the arms slightly forward to release.

Isolation Movements and Static Stretches

1. *Shoulder rotations*

    a. With arms down at your sides, press your shoulders forward, up toward the ears, back, and then relax them down. Repeat 8 times.

    b. Reverse the movement by pressing the shoulders back, up toward the ears, forward, and then relax them down. Repeat 8 times.

2. *Neck stretch and head rolls*

    a. Tilt your head to the right, moving your right ear toward your right shoulder.

    b. Gently drop your chin toward your chest and roll your head to the left, making a half-circle.

    c. Return your head to an upright position.

    d. Reverse the movement by tilting your head to the left and continuing the half-circle motion to the right.

    e. Return to the starting position and repeat 4 times.

3. *Back stretch*

    a. Place your feet shoulder-distance apart, bend your knees slightly, and release the hips back. Tilt your

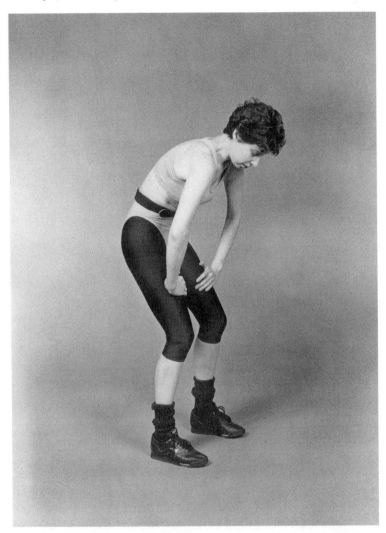

torso forward and place your hands on your thighs for
support. Inhale.

b. Exhale on the count of four and gently tilt the pelvis
forward to stretch your lower back.

c. Return to the starting position and repeat 4 times.

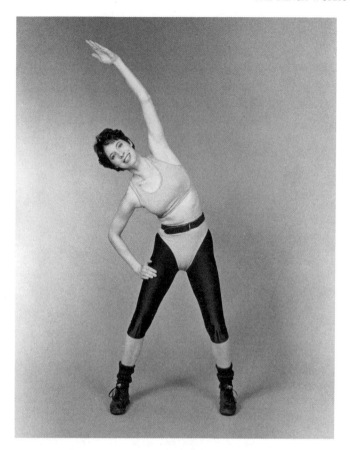

4. *Torso stretch*
   a. Place your feet shoulder-distance apart and bend your knees slightly. Lift your left arm to the ceiling and place your right hand on the outside of your right thigh for support. Inhale.
   b. Exhale and tilt your torso to the right. You will feel a stretch in the left side of your torso. Breathe steadily as you hold this position for 10 to 20 seconds.
   c. Return to an upright position, change arms, and repeat to the other side.

5. *Calf stretch—variation 1*

    a. Standing in a lunge position, with hands at your waist, bend your right knee and extend your left leg back. Your body will describe a long diagonal from the left heel to your head. Both feet should be pointed forward, and the left heel raised slightly.

    b. Press your left heel toward the floor. Hold the stretch for 10 to 20 seconds.

    c. Repeat with your right leg extended back.

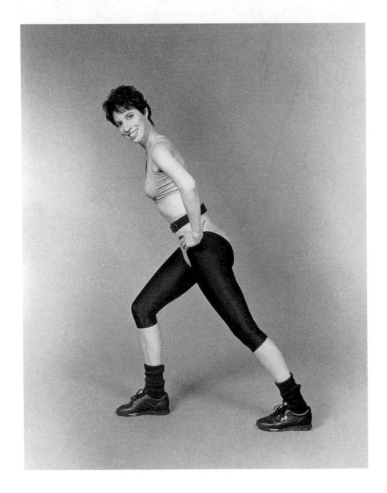

Variation 2

  a. Stand with your right leg placed slightly in front of the left leg. Both feet should be pointing forward.

  b. Bend both knees until you feel a stretch in the left calf. Breathe steadily as you hold the position for 10 to 20 seconds.

  c. Reverse legs and repeat the stretch.

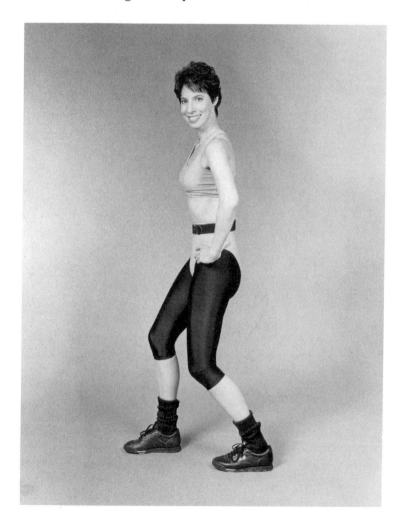

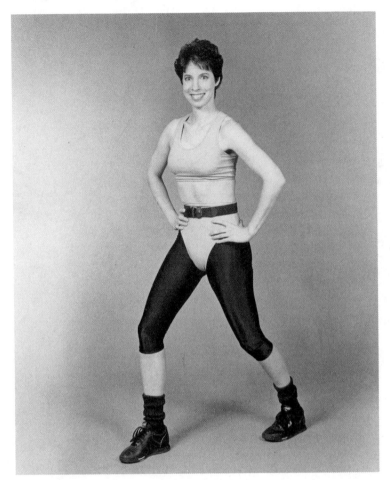

6. *Hip flexor stretch*
   a. Position your legs as in variation 1 of the calf stretch, with hands at your waist.
   b. Tilt your pelvis forward until you feel a stretch in the front of your left hip. (Hold your torso perpendicular to the floor for this stretch.) Breathe steadily and hold the position for 10 to 20 seconds.
   c. Reverse legs and repeat the stretch.

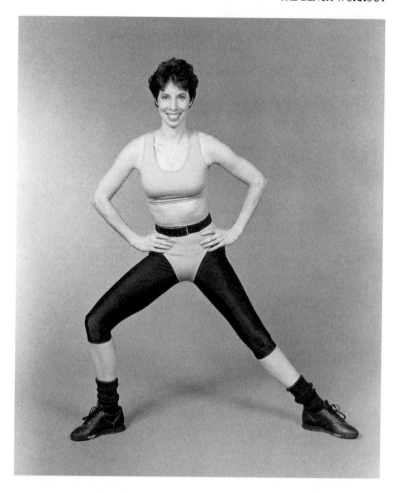

7. *Inner thigh stretch*
   a. Separate your legs wide with your feet turned out on a diagonal.
   b. Bend the right knee (make sure your knee is aligned over the center of your right foot), and hold the stretch for 10 to 20 seconds.
   c. Return to the starting position and repeat to the left side.

8. *Hamstring stretch*

    a. Place the right foot in front of the left foot, and bend the left knee. Tilt your hips back so that your torso describes a diagonal in space, and flex the right foot. Place your hands on your left thigh for support. Hold the position for 10 to 20 seconds.

    b. Change sides and repeat.

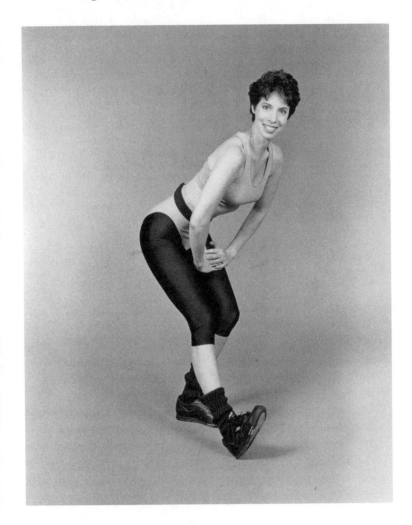

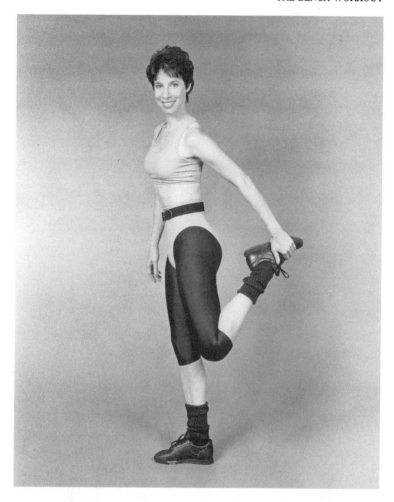

9. *Quadriceps stretch*
  a. Standing on your right leg, bend your left leg behind
      you and clasp the instep with your left hand. If
      necessary, hold onto a chair for balance.
  b. Press your foot into your hand and hold the stretch
      for 10 to 20 seconds.
  c. Change legs and repeat to the other side.

5

BODY MECHANICS GUIDELINES FOR "DOING THE BENCH RIGHT"

IMPORTANT: *Read this before proceeding to exercise.*

While the Bench Workout is easy to learn and perform, stepping up and down on a platform with hand-held weights demands that the exerciser have an awareness of body placement and alignment. Following the guidelines suggested below will help ensure a workout that is safe as well as effective.

POSTURE AND BENCH-STEPPING TECHNIQUE TIPS

- Stand tall with your shoulders in line with your hips, your abdominals lifted, and your tailbone dropped (no arched backs).
- As you step up and down on the bench try to keep from leaning forward at the hips, as this places too much strain on the lower back. Instead, use a full body lean when stepping on and off the bench.

- Your knee should bend no farther than a 90-degree angle when you raise your foot to step onto the bench and back off. An angle sharper than 90 degrees will place undue stress on the knee joint.

- When stepping on or off the bench, use your entire foot. Place the ball of the foot down, then "roll" your foot until the heel touches. Neglecting to lower your heel to contact the bench or floor will shorten and contract the calf muscles. By touching the heel down firmly with each step, you prompt the muscle to elongate.

- Knees should never lock in the stepping action. Concentrate on keeping your knee joints relaxed.

- Always be aware of where you're stepping; keep an eye on the bench.

- Never step forward off the bench (as when stepping down stairs). The stepping action in this position places too much stress on the knee.

- Practice the foot patterns before adding the upper body motions.

- Sometimes doing a new repetitive exercise can make you feel disoriented. That is normal. If you ever feel disoriented while bench stepping, get off the bench and march in place until you feel more comfortable.

- Don't forget proper body mechanics when lifting and carrying your bench. Remember to bend your knees when you lift the bench, and be sure to hold the bench close to you (not at arm's length) when carrying it.

USING WEIGHTS CORRECTLY

- Hold the hand weights securely, but not tightly. An overly tight grip can create a rise in blood pressure.
- Arm movements should be executed in a slow and controlled manner. Never swing the weights, as the force of momentum can take the limb beyond its normal range of motion.
- Your elbow joints should never lock when performing the upper body movements. When you extend your arms, keep a slight looseness in the elbows.
- Never warm up with weights. The warm-up is designed to prepare the muscles and joints for more vigorous activity. Remember that a warm-up is not a workout and that adding weight resistance before your muscles are sufficiently limber is potentially harmful.
- Do not use weights until you are familiar with and comfortable with the arm movements.

NOTE: Some individuals should not use weights. *Do not use weights* if you are hypertensive, have joint or orthopedic problems, are more than three months pregnant, or are significantly overweight.

6

THE BENCH WORKOUT

The Bench Workout is divided into three parts: Part I consists of eight basic bench-stepping movements, Part II combines these movements into two routines for a twenty-minute aerobic workout, and Part III gives you instructions for an aerobic cool-down.

As you learn the basic movements keep the following points in mind:

- Before you begin any of the basic steps, be sure to read through all the directions for the movement. Then execute the leg motions in isolation, *before* you add the arm movements. Keep your hands occupied by placing them at your waist while you learn the leg actions.
- Make sure your legs are getting a balanced workout. As the leg that leads the movement gets more of a workout than the follower, you'll need to structure the routine so that your legs get equal time. You can perform the basic movements in two ways: (a) you can alternate the leg that starts the pattern each time you perform the movement, or (b) you can repeat a series of movements starting with one leg, then switch to the other leg to begin the movement for an equivalent series. If you choose the latter routine, do

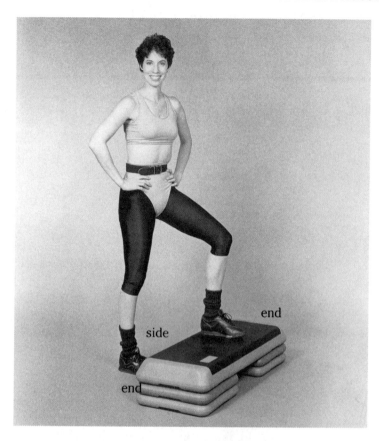

not lead with the same leg for more than a minute. After one minute (or less), repeat the movement an equal number of times, now leading with the other leg.

- When stepping up and down from the bench, some exercisers have a tendency to stomp on the landing surface. Try to place your foot lightly to eliminate a stress-impact force on the lower leg.
- You can approach the bench from different directions. You may want to create some of your own steps, but remember not to step *forward off* the bench (so that you finish with your back to the bench).

PART I—THE BENCH-STEPPING MOVEMENTS

The Basic "Up-Down"

Starting position: Stand with your feet together facing the side of the bench. Place your hands at your waist.

1. March in place for 8 counts (1 count equals 1 step) on the floor, starting with the right foot.

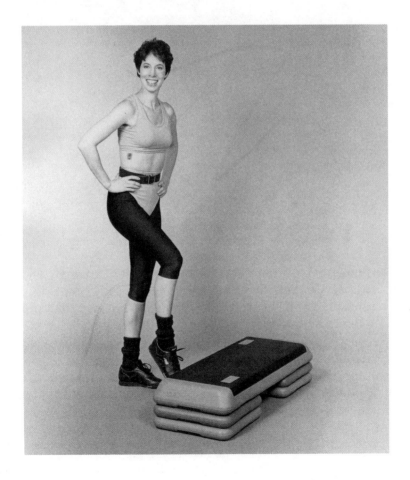

2. Step up on the bench, starting with the right foot, and march 8 counts on the bench.

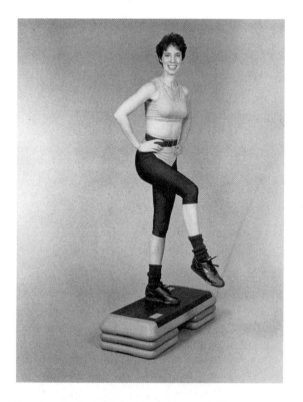

3. Step back off the bench with the right foot first, and march 4 counts on the floor.

4. Step up on the bench with the right foot and march 4 counts on the bench.

5. Step back off the bench with the right foot and march 2 counts on the floor.

6. Step up on the bench with the right foot and march 2 counts on the bench. Repeat the 2-counts variation seven more times.

Movements 1–6 equal one cycle.

To begin the series again, this time starting with the left foot, you perform a "tap" step.*

1. As your left foot lands on the bench at the last of the 2-counts variation, instead of placing your entire foot down, tap the ball of your foot on the bench.

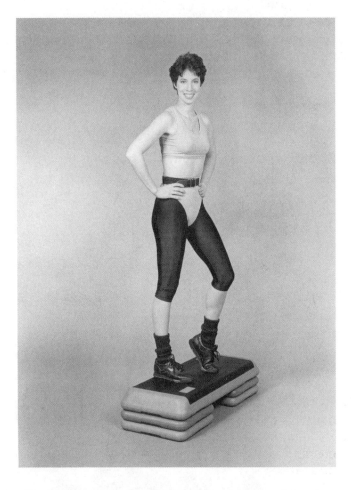

*Note: The "tap" step can be used throughout the various bench-stepping movements to enable you to change the leg that starts the pattern.

2. Then, with the same foot, step down on the floor and march in place for 8 counts.

The remainder of the series will be performed with your left foot leading.

Arm variation:
You can pump your arms forward and back at your sides, with elbows bent, throughout the series. When your right leg is lifted your left arm should be slightly forward, and vice versa when your left leg is lifted.

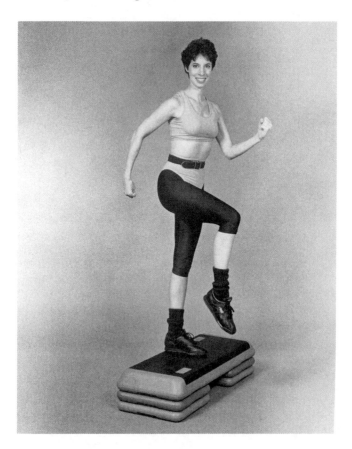

The Knee Lift with Biceps Curl

Starting position: Stand with your feet together, facing the side of the bench, with arms down at your sides.

1. Step up on the bench with your right foot.

2. Lift your left knee as you bend your elbows, bringing your palms toward your shoulders.

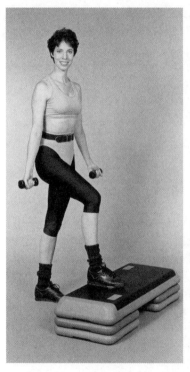 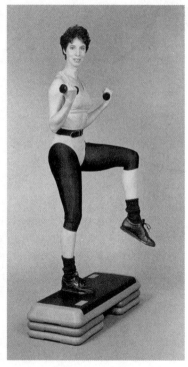

3. Step back off the bench with your left foot, lowering your arms to your sides.
4. Place your right foot on the floor.

Movements 1–4 equal one cycle.

To continue the movement alternating sides . . .

5. Step up on the bench with your left foot, arms at your sides.
6. Lift your right knee as you bring palms up toward your shoulders.
7. Step back off the bench with your right foot, lowering your arms to your sides.
8. Place your left foot on the floor.

This movement can be performed with one leg leading continually by adding the tap step on the fourth count (number 4 above). Instead of placing your right foot on the floor, tap the ball of your foot. Your right foot is then ready to lead the series again.

The V Step

Starting position: Stand with your feet together, facing the side of the bench, arms down at your sides.

1. Step up on the bench with your right foot slightly to the right of center of the bench. Simultaneously raise your right arm above your head on an upward right diagonal (making one side of a V).
2. Step up on the bench with your left foot slightly to the left of the center, creating a straddle position. Raise your left arm above your head on an upward left diagonal, completing the V.

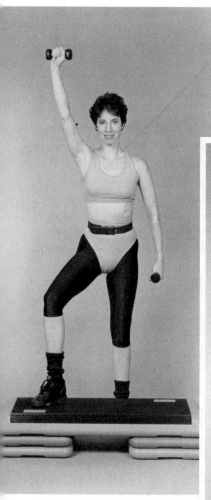

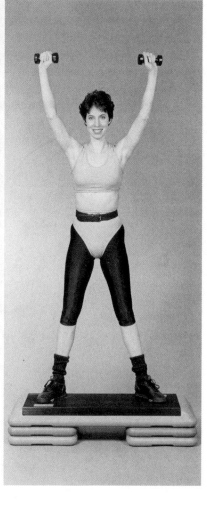

3. Step back off the bench with your right foot and lower your right arm down.

4. Step back off the bench with your left foot and lower your left arm down.

Movements 1–4 equal one cycle.

This movement will continue with your right leg leading until you perform a tap step to change sides. To change sides, tap your left foot on number 4 and then begin the series with the left foot.

Arm variation:
Instead of lifting and lowering one arm at a time, raise both arms up as your right foot steps up on the bench. Keep both arms lifted as your left foot steps up on the bench. Lower both arms as the right foot and then the left foot step back off the bench.

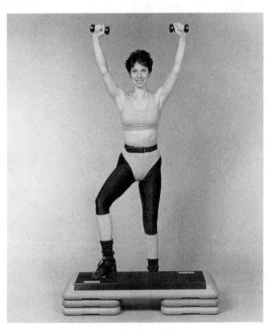

Hamstring Curl with Lateral Arm Pull

Starting position: Stand with feet together, facing the side of the bench, your arms down at your sides.

1. Step up on the bench with your right foot slightly turned out, angling your body to the right.

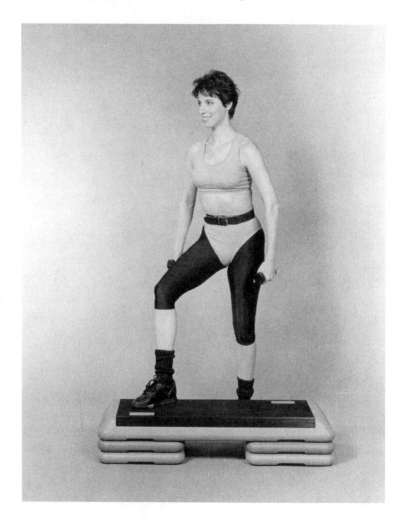

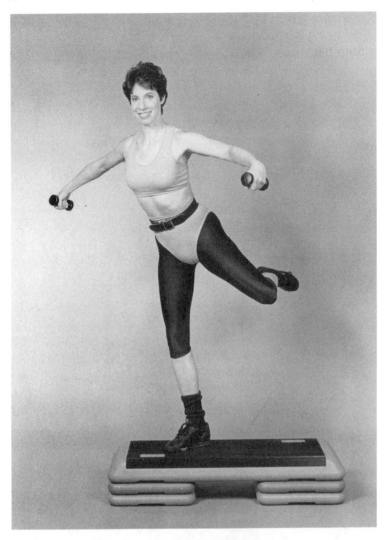

2. Bend your left knee, bringing your heel toward your left buttock. You should be leaning slightly forward. (Make sure your abdominals are working—do not let your back arch.) Simultaneously pull your arms out to the sides up to about shoulder height.

3. Step back off the bench with your left foot and return arms to your sides.

4. Step back off the bench with your right foot.

Movements 1–4 equal one cycle.

To continue the movement, alternating sides . . .

5. Step up on the bench with your left foot slightly turned out, angling your body to the left.

6. Bend your right knee as in number 2.

7. Step back off the bench with your right leg and return your arms to your sides.

8. Step back off the bench with your left leg.

If you want to perform this movement repeatedly leading with the same leg, simply add the tap step on the fourth count (number 4 above). Instead of placing your right foot on the floor, tap the ball of your foot. The right foot is then ready to lead the series again.

Traveling Side Knee Lift with Forward Arm Press

Starting position: Stand with your feet together, facing the side of the bench, with arms down at your sides.

1. Angling your body slightly to the right, step up to the far right corner of the bench with your left foot. Hold your hands in front of your shoulders, with palms forward.

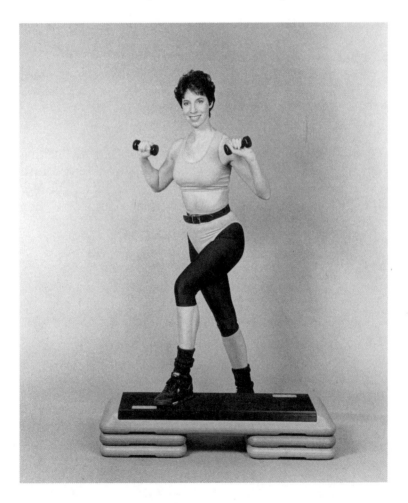

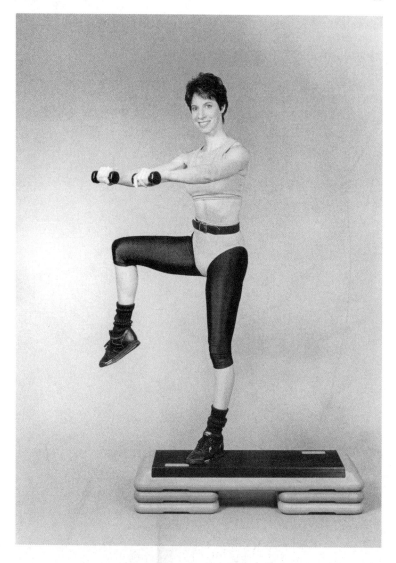

2. Lift your right knee up to the side as you press both arms forward.
3. Step back off the bench with your right foot and bring your hands back to your shoulders.

4. Place your left foot on the floor, separating your legs at least shoulder distance apart. Hands remain at your shoulders.

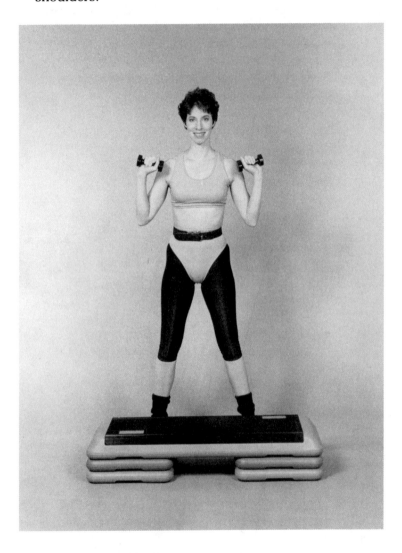

Movements 1–4 equal one cycle.

To continue the movement but alternating sides . . .

5. Angling your body slightly to the left, step up to the left corner of the bench with your right foot. Hold your hands in front of your shoulders.
6. Lift your left knee up to the side as you press both arms forward.
7. Step back off the bench with your left foot and bring your hands back to your shoulders.
8. Place your right foot on the floor, separating your legs at least shoulder-distance apart. Hands remain at your shoulders.

To perform this movement with one leg leading in a series, add the tap step on the fourth count (number 4). Your left foot is then ready to lead the series again.

Side Leg Lift with Pulley-Action Arms

Starting position: Stand with your feet together, facing the side of the bench, your arms down at your sides.

1. Angling your body slightly to the right, step up to the far right corner of the bench with your left foot. Hold your arms stretched down in front of your body, with your hands in a fist and close together.

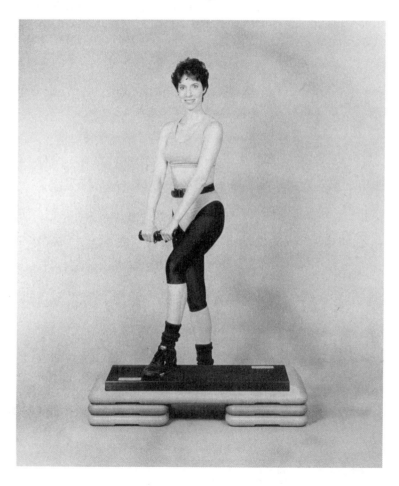

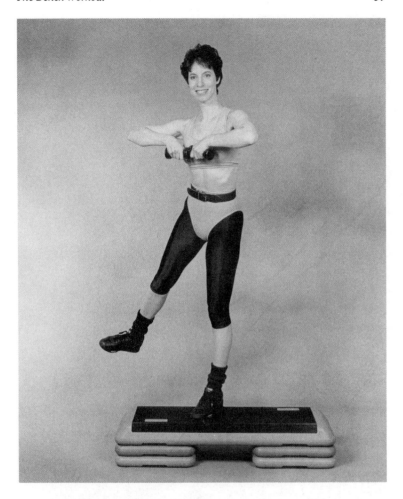

2. Lift your right leg slightly up to the side, trying not to lift your hip. (It helps to think of pushing your foot down before lifting your leg.) Simultaneously pull your hands up to your breastbone (elbows will bend out to the sides), simulating the action of a pulley. Shoulders should not lift during the arm action.

3. Step back off the bench with your right foot and push arms back down to lengthened position.

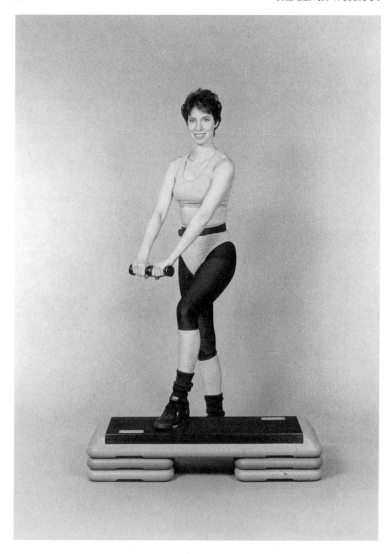

4. Place your left foot on the floor, separating your legs at least shoulder distance apart. Arms remain down.

Movements 1–4 equal one cycle.

To continue, alternating sides . . .

5. Angling your body slightly to the left, step up to the left corner of the bench with your right foot.
6. Lift your left leg up to the side as you pull your hands up to your breastbone.
7. Step back off the bench with your left foot and extend your arms down to their full length.
8. Place your right foot on the floor.

To perform this movement with one leg leading in a series, add the tap step on the fourth count (number 4). Your left foot is then ready to lead the series again.

The Bench Straddle with Triceps Extension

Starting position: Stand with your feet together, facing one end of the bench, with arms down at your sides.

1. Step up on the bench with your right foot. Bend your elbows and place your arms slightly behind your torso, with forearms at rib level.

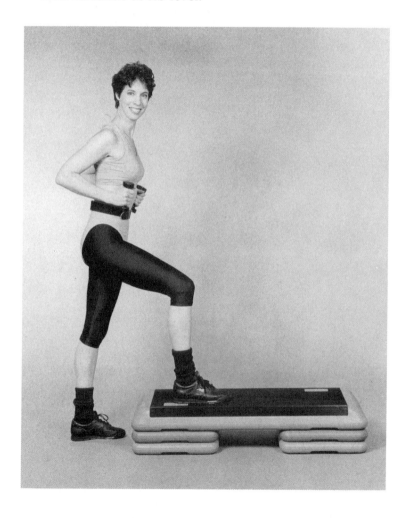

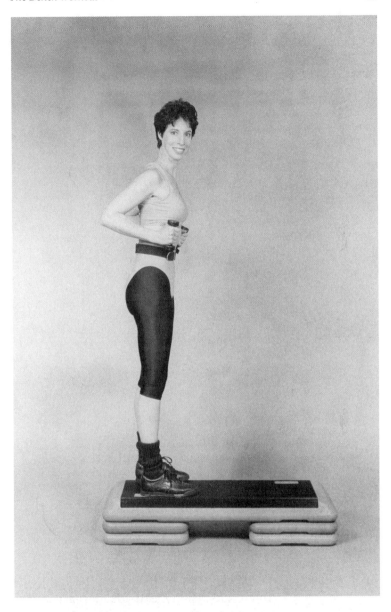

2. Step up on the bench with your left foot.

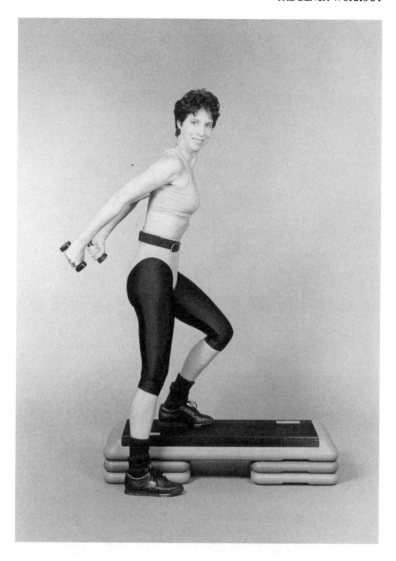

3. Place your right foot down on the floor on the right side of the bench. Simultaneously extend your forearms back (straightening your arms); try to keep your elbows stationary.

4. Straddle the bench by placing your left foot down on the floor on the left side of the bench. Your arms should remain extended back.

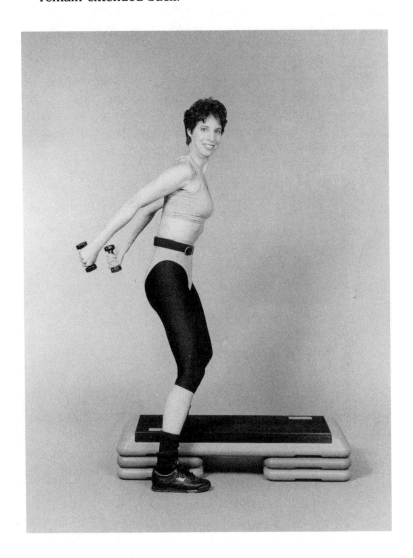

Movements 1–4 equal one cycle.

To continue, repeating the movement with the right leg leading . . .

5. Step up on the bench with your right foot and bend your elbows (same as movement 1).
6. Repeat movements 2, 3, and 4.

The movement series can be performed with the left leg starting the pattern with a tap step on the fourth count (movement 4 above). Instead of placing your left foot on the floor, tap the ball of your foot. Now your left foot is ready to step up on the bench and begin the series.

The Lunge Back with Forward Punch

Starting position: Approaching the bench from the side, step onto it at one end, placing feet together and facing the other end. Place your heels toward the edge of the bench. With elbows bent, hold both hands in front of your shoulders, palms out.

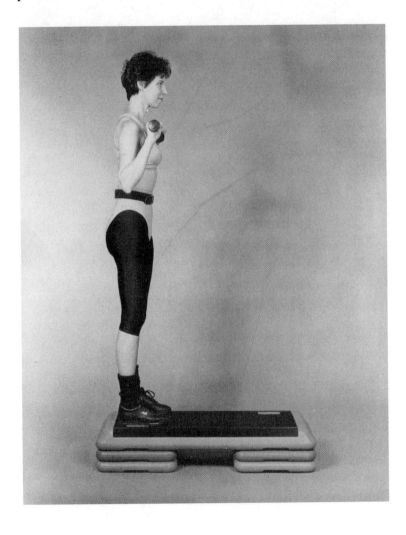

1. Lunge your right leg back, putting your right foot on the floor but keeping your weight on the left. Simultaneously punch your right arm forward. Your body will describe a long diagonal in space.

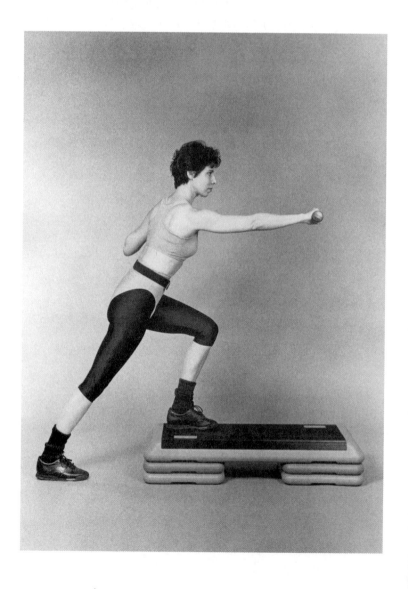

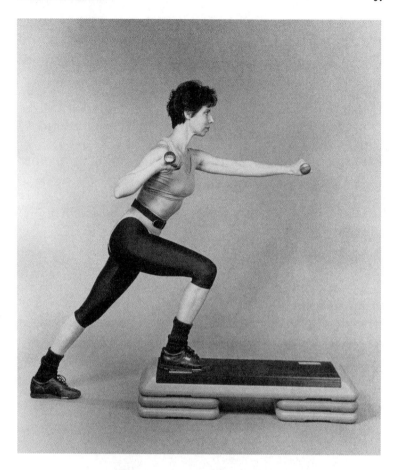

2. Return your right foot to the bench and your right hand to your shoulder (as in the starting position).
3. Lunge your left leg back, putting your left foot on the floor but keeping your weight on the right. Simultaneously punch your left arm forward.
4. Return your left foot to the bench and your left hand to your shoulder.

Movements 1–4 equal one cycle.

Continue alternating legs or do a variation of this exercise by repeating the lunge back three times on one leg before alternating legs. To repeat . . .

1. Lunge back as in number 1 above.
2. Return your right foot to the bench with a tap instead of placing weight on that foot. Your right hand returns to your shoulder.
3. Lunge back again with the right leg and give another right-arm punch.
4. Repeat the tap step.
5. Lunge back again with the right leg and repeat the right-arm punch.
6. Return your right foot to the bench.
7. Transfer your weight to the right foot and lunge back with your left leg.

Arm variation:
Instead of punching one arm forward as your leg lunges back, punch with both arms.

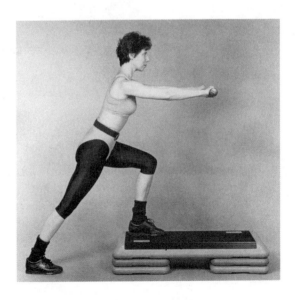

PART II—THE ROUTINES

The eight bench-stepping movements have been coordinated into two ten-minute routines that make up the twenty-minute aerobic Bench Workout. Before jumping (or, more precisely, stepping) into these routines, take a few minutes to look over the sequence of movements. A variation for the arms is provided occasionally, and there are instructions for transitional movements to help lead you smoothly from one pattern to the next.

As you execute the routines, it is essential that you "listen" to the signals your body gives you. If you begin to feel breathless or it is difficult for you to speak, you are working too hard. Decrease the level of intensity: Put down the hand weights, stop using your arms, or get off the bench and perform the movements on the floor.

You do not have to complete both routines or even one routine. Remember the principle of progression. Do what you can and gradually increase the length of time you do it.

It is important that you monitor your heart rate while doing the routines. You may want to take your pulse every five or six minutes to check if you're in your training zone.

ROUTINE 1

NOTE: The routines have been worked out so that the legs alternate properly. Just follow the directions and you will be ready to start each consecutive movement with the correct leg.

Movement	**Approximate Duration**

1. *The Basic Up-Down*

    a. With hands on your waist, lead off with your right leg. Repeat the complete cycle twice; finish with a tap step on the last count (the tap step is performed on the bench).   60 seconds total

    b. With your arms pumping, start the march on the bench with your left leg. Repeat the complete cycle twice, then finish with a tap step on the last count (the tap step is performed on the floor).   60 seconds total

2. *Knee lift with biceps curls*

    a. With hands on your waist, lead off with your right leg and alternate legs for 16 cycles.   60 seconds total

    b. Add biceps curls with your arms and continue the leg movements for another 16 cycles. Tap step on the last count.

3. *Traveling side leg lift with pulley action*

    a. With hands on your waist, lead off with your left leg and alternate legs for 16 cycles.   60 seconds total

Movement	**Approximate Duration**

   b. Add arm movements and continue the leg movements for another 16 cycles. Tap step on the last count.

4. *Transition*
With hands on your waist and leading with your right leg, start a march on the floor for 32 counts. Move toward the end of the bench in preparation for the bench straddle.   15 seconds total

5. *The bench straddle with triceps extensions*
   a. With hands on your waist and the right leg leading, step up on the bench to begin 16 cycles of the pattern. Tap step on the last count.   75 seconds total
   b. Add arm movements as the left leg starts for 16 cycles. Tap step on the last count.

6. *Transition*
With hands on your waist and the right leg leading, begin a march on the bench for 32 counts.   15 seconds total

Movement	Approximate Duration

7. *The lunge back with forward punch and bench straddle*

   a. With hands on your waist and the right leg leading, begin the lunge back for 4 cycles.

   b. Add arm movements as the right leg starts the lunge back for 4 additional cycles.

15 seconds total (for a and b)

   c. Keeping your hands on your waist, perform the bench straddle with your right leg leading for 4 cycles. (Remember that you start on top of the bench and the movement begins with a step down to the right side of the bench.)

   d. Add arm movements as the right leg continues to lead the bench straddle for 4 more cycles.

15 seconds total (for c and d)

   e. Repeat "b" for 4 cycles.

30 seconds total (for e, f, g, h)

   f. Repeat "d" for 4 cycles.

   g. Repeat "b" for 4 cycles.

   h. Repeat "d" for 4 cycles. Tap step on the last count.

Now put your hands on your waist. Starting with your left leg, march on the bench for 32 counts.

15 seconds total

Movement	Approximate Duration

i. With your left leg leading, repeat the entire sequence (a through h). — 60 seconds total

8. *Transition*
With hands on your waist and beginning with your right leg, march on the bench for 32 counts. Step back off the bench with your right leg again leading, and march for 16 counts on the floor to the front of the bench in preparation for the V step. — 25 seconds total

9. *The V step*
a. With hands on your waist and beginning with your right leg, perform 16 cycles. Tap step on the last count. — 30 seconds total

b. With hands still on your waist, lead off with the left leg for 16 cycles. Tap step on the last count. — 30 seconds total

c. Add the arm movement, now leading off with the right leg for 16 cycles. Tap step on the last count. — 30 seconds total

d. Continue using your arms, and lead off with your left leg for another 16 cycles. Tap step on the last count. — 30 seconds total

Movement	Approximate Duration

10. *Transition*
Keeping your hands on your
waist, march in place for 32
counts.   15 seconds total

Total Duration: 10 minutes, 25 seconds

Congratulations on completing the first routine! Remember, you can stop here and gradually increase the length of time you spend exercising in future workouts. If you're ready to challenge your endurance ability, then continue with Routine 2.

ROUTINE 2

Movement	Approximate duration

1. *The basic up-down*
  a. With hands on your waist,
lead off with your right
leg. Repeat the complete
cycle twice; finish with a
tap step on the last count
(the tap step is performed
on the bench).   60 seconds total
  b. With your arms pumping
and leading with the left
leg, begin a march on the
bench. Repeat the complete cycle twice. (This
cycle starts with 8 marches

Movement   **Approximate Duration**

on the bench, followed by 8 marches on the floor, and so on.) On the last count of the second cycle, your right foot should land on the floor (with no tap step).   60 seconds total

2. *Traveling side knee lift with forward arm press*
   a. With hands on your waist, step up on the bench with your left leg to begin 16 alternating cycles.   30 seconds total
   b. Add the arm movements and with your left leg step up on bench to begin another 16 alternating cycles. Tap step on the last count.   30 seconds total

3. *Knee lift with biceps curl*
   a. With hands on your waist and leading with your right leg, step up onto the bench to begin the knee-lift pattern. Tap step on the last count of the first cycle. Repeat the cycle 7 more times, leading off with the right leg each time.   30 seconds total (for a and b)
   b. Add the arm movements and repeat the cycle with

Movement	Approximate Duration

your right leg leading off
8 times. On the last count
of cycle 8, place your right
foot on the floor (no tap
step).

c. With hands on your waist
and leading with your left
leg, step up onto the
bench to begin the knee-
lift pattern. Tap step on
the last count of the first
cycle. Repeat the cycle 7
more times, always lead-   30 seconds total (for
ing with your left leg.   c and d)

d. Add the arm movements
and repeat the cycle with
your left leg leading 8
times. On the last count
of cycle 8 place your left
foot on the floor (no tap
step).

4. *Transition*

   a. With hands on your waist,
lead off with your right
leg to start a march on
the floor for 32 counts.   30 seconds total

   b. Place your hands in front
of your shoulders, stretch
your arms up to the ceil-
ing, and return your hands
to your shoulders as you
continue to march for 32
counts.

Movement	Approximate Duration
5. *Hamstring curl with lateral arm pull*	
a. With hands on your waist, step up onto the bench with your right foot to begin the hamstring curl pattern. Tap step on the last count of the first cycle. Repeat the cycle 7 more times, always starting with the right leg.	30 seconds total (for a and b)
b. Add the arm movements and repeat the cycle with your right leg starting 8 times. On the last count of cycle 8, place your right foot on the floor (no tap step).	
c. With hands on your waist, step up onto bench with your left leg to begin the hamstring curl pattern. Tap step on the last count of the first cycle. Repeat the cycle 7 more times, always starting with the left leg.	30 seconds total (for c and d)
d. Add the arm movements and repeat the cycle 8 times, with your left leg starting each time. On the last count of cycle 8, place your left foot on the floor (no tap step).	

Movement	Approximate Duration

e. Using your arms, alternate the pattern for 16 cycles. Your right leg starts cycle 1.   30 seconds total

6. *The V step*
  a. With hands on your waist, lead off with your right leg for 16 cycles. Tap step on the last count.   30 seconds total
  b. Moving both arms, lead off with your left leg for 16 cycles. Tap step on the last count.   30 seconds total

7. *Transition*
With hands on your waist and leading with your right leg, start a march on the floor for 32 counts. March toward the end of the bench in preparation for the bench straddle.   15 seconds total

8. *The bench straddle with triceps extension*
  a. With hands on your waist and leading with your right leg, step up on the bench to begin 16 cycles of the pattern. Tap step on the last count.   75 seconds total
  b. Add the arm movements and, leading with your left

Movement	**Approximate Duration**
leg, perform 16 cycles of the exercise. Tap step on the last count.	

9. *Transition*
    a. With hands on your waist and leading with your right leg, march on the bench for 16 counts.   15 seconds total
    b. With hands still on your waist, lead with your right leg back off the bench. March on the floor to the side of the bench in 16 counts.

10. *The V step*
    Repeat sequence 6.   60 seconds total

Total duration: 9 minutes, 45 seconds

PART III—THE COOL-DOWN

After performing the routines, it's essential you complete the workout with an aerobic cool-down. *Do not stop abruptly* after you've finished the cardiovascular portion of this program. By taking just three to five minutes for a cool-down, you'll gradually lower your heart rate and prevent blood from pooling in the lower extremities.

In the cool-down, you'll want to decrease the intensity of the workout gradually. Begin by stepping off the bench. You can march in place for a minute and then repeat one or two of the bench-stepping movements on the floor for another minute. You might want to try the V step or hamstring curl without the arm movements. Next, take a slow walk around the room.

After three or four minutes, check your pulse for a recovery heart rate. If your heart rate is not below 120 beats per minute, continue walking slowly until it drops to that level.

You can finish the cool-down with one to two minutes of some of the same isolation movements and static stretches that make up the warm-up. The back stretch, torso stretch, calf stretch, hip flexor stretch, inner thigh stretch, hamstring stretch, and quadriceps stretch will help lengthen muscles that were contracted during the routines. Include the shoulder rotations, the neck stretch, and head rolls if your neck and shoulders feel tight. Also, try some of the flexibility exercises in chapter 7.

7

STRENGTHEN AND STRETCH ON THE BENCH

T he beauty of the bench is its adaptability. Not only can you get a great aerobic workout by stepping up and down on it, but you can also use the bench for strength training and stretching. Use your bench creatively to complete your workout with muscle-conditioning and flexibility exercises.

On some days you may just want to do the strengthening and stretching exercises and skip the aerobic work. That's fine, but remember that the warm-up should also be performed prior to these exercises.

MUSCLE STRENGTHENING

Strengthening exercises tone and define your muscles and enable you to do more work without becoming fatigued. Many of the exercises in this section can be done with weights to "overload" the muscles. Don't worry about creating excessive bulk—that's the result of rigorous body-building and heavy weight training. (In fact, most women will never develop bulky muscles. The male hormone, testosterone, which is responsible for the greater muscle mass in men, is limited in females.)

We'll focus on the muscle groups of the abdomen and upper body in these exercises, since we worked the lower body intensely throughout the aerobic portion of the workout. The exercises are presented in repetitions and sets. A set is comprised of ten repetitions, and it's recommended that you try to accomplish two or three sets of each exercise. After each set, take a moment to rest before starting the next series of repetitions.

The overload and progression principles, both described in chapter 2, are important here. You should try to perform two or three sets of an exercise before using weights or adding more weight. Add weight in increments of one pound for each hand. Once your muscles have adapted to the sets (meaning that you are able to do all the repetitions), add more weight. You won't use weights for either the abdomen or the triceps push-up exercises.

Before beginning, you may want to place a towel or blanket on your bench to make it more comfortable.

Bench Press

This exercise works the pectorals (chest) and deltoids (shoulders).

Starting position: Lie face-up on the bench. Bend your knees, and if the bench is long enough, place both feet on the bench. Otherwise, place your feet on the floor. Throughout the exercise, be sure to press your lower back into the bench. *Do not let your back arch.*

1. Position your arms with elbows out to the side and forearms and hands raised perpendicular to the floor. Inhale.

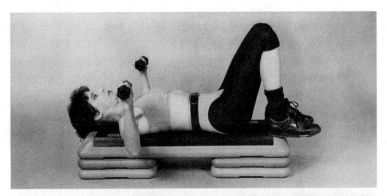

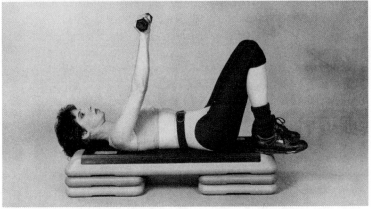

2. Exhale and extend your arms up to the ceiling over your chest.
3. Inhale and return your arms to position 1.
4. Exhale and repeat movement 2. Continue your repetitions.

Remember, try to perform 10 repetitions (one set), rest, and complete one or two more sets for this exercise and the other muscle-strengthening exercises.

Bent-Arm Flyes

Flyes strengthen the pectoral muscles.

Starting position: Same as for the bench press.

1. Hold your arms with elbows out to your sides and hands extended farther out to either side and palms facing in. Inhale.

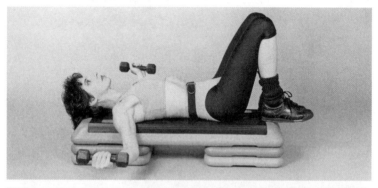

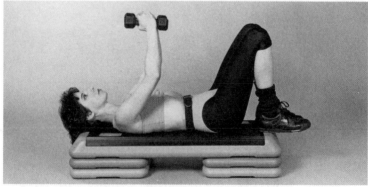

2. Exhale and extend your arms up to the ceiling over chest. (Your arms will not straighten completely.)
3. Inhale and return the arms to position 1.
4. Exhale and repeat movement 2. Continue your repetitions.

Upper Back Strengthener

This exercise works the trapezius and rhomboid muscles located in the middle of the upper back.

Starting position: Lying on your stomach with knees bent, pull in your abdominals and tilt your pelvis slightly forward to prevent your back from arching.

1. Extend your arms out to your sides at shoulder level, keeping elbows slightly bent. Inhale.

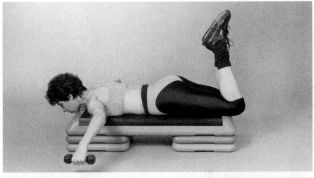

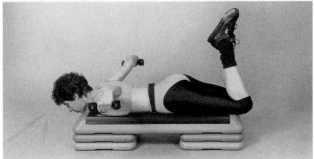

2. Exhale and lift your arms straight up. (You will feel your shoulder blades pulling together as you lift your arms.)
3. Inhale and return your arms to position 1.
4. Exhale and repeat movement 2. Continue repetitions.

Concentration Curls

Curls work the biceps (the front of your upper arms).

Starting position: Sit on the bench with your legs separated and feet on the floor.

1. Place your left hand on your left thigh for support. Extend your right arm down to the floor; rest the back of the right arm against the inside of your right thigh. Inhale.

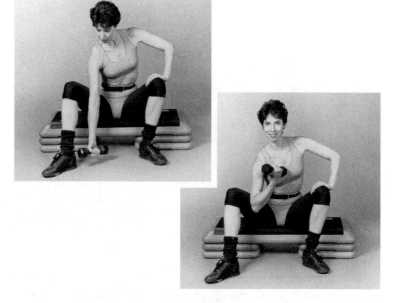

2. Exhale. Keeping the elbow stationary, bend your right arm and raise your forearm, bringing the palm of your hand to the breastbone.
3. Inhale and return arm to position 1.
4. Exhale and repeat movement 2. Continue your repetitions. After completing sets with the right arm, repeat the exercise with your left arm.

Triceps Push-ups

These will help strengthen the back of the upper arms.

Starting position: Sitting in front of the bench with your hips close to the bench, bend your knees and place feet on floor.

1. Place your hands palms down on the edge of the bench with your fingers facing forward. Keep your elbows close to your sides (they should not flare out). Inhale.

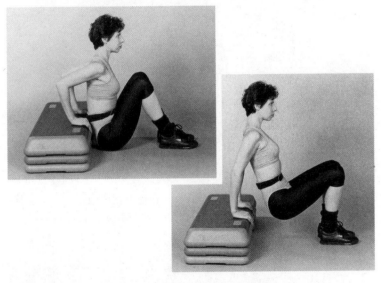

2. Exhale and press your palms against the bench to straighten your arms. Your hips will lift from the floor.
3. Inhale and bend your elbows, but do *not* rest your hips on the floor.
4. Exhale and repeat movement 2. Continue repetitions.

NOTE: If you find it too difficult to perform the triceps push-up using the bench, you can do this exercise with your palms on the floor.

Crunches

Crunches condition the abdominal muscles.

Starting position: Lying on your back on the floor, bend your knees and place your feet close together on the bench. Press your lower back into the floor.

1. Place your hands behind your head. Inhale.

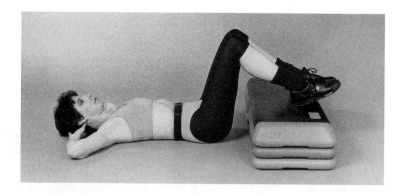

2. Exhale and pull in your abdominal muscles as you lift your shoulder blades off the floor. (Make sure you keep elbows to the side.)

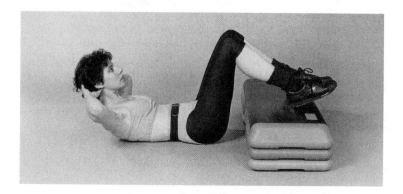

3. Inhale and return the torso to position 1 but do not lower your shoulders all the way to the floor. Keep the torso slightly raised.

4. Exhale and repeat movement 2. Continue repetitions.

Variation

As you lift your shoulder blades off the floor, rotate your torso to the right. Alternate sides.

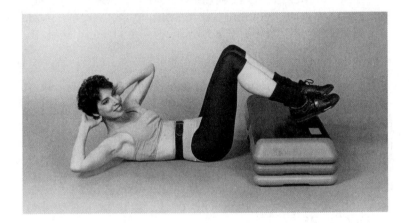

MUSCLE FLEXIBILITY

Stretching exercises not only make you feel good, they're also good for you. Stretching elongates the muscles, ligaments, and tendons and is particularly important after muscle-strengthening and aerobic work. Muscles contract during the workout and flexibility exercises help restore length to the muscle fibers. Slow stretching is also a great way to release tension and relax.

The stretches in this section target the specific muscle groups that have been contracted during the aerobic workout and strength-training program. As you stretch, keep the following points in mind:

- Do not hold your breath. Exhale deeply as you position your body into the stretch, and then breathe naturally as you hold the stretch.
- Do not bounce to increase the stretch. Bouncing or ballistic movements strain the muscles and can tear muscle fibers. A static stretch (holding the position) will effectively lengthen the muscles and connective tissues.
- To stretch a muscle most effectively, hold the position for ten to thirty seconds.

Calf Stretch

1. Stand on the bench with your right foot flat to support your weight. (It is best if you stand in the middle of the bench lengthwise for stability.) Place the arch of your left foot on the edge of the bench, letting the heel hang down. Bending your right leg slightly, place your weight on the left foot. Hold the stretch.
2. Change legs and repeat.

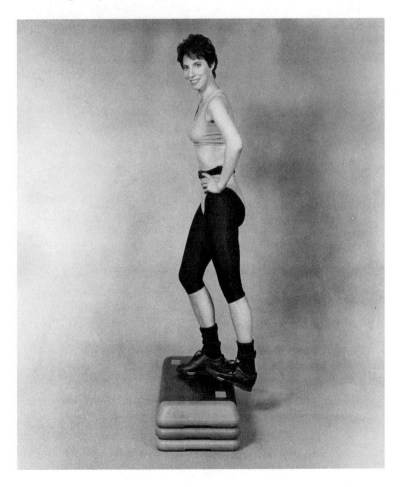

Hip Flexor Stretch

1. Lying on your back lengthwise on the bench, hug your right knee to your chest. Extend your left leg forward so that only your left heel touches the floor. Hold the stretch.
2. Change legs and repeat.

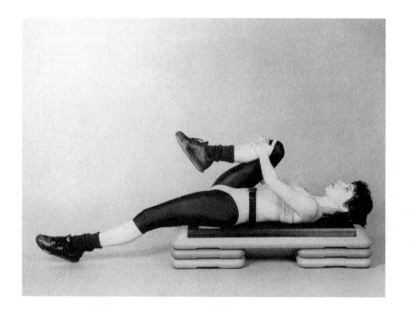

Hamstring Stretch

1. Lying on your back lengthwise on the bench, bend your left knee and place your left foot on the bench. Extend your right leg to the ceiling and, with your hands on the back of your thigh, gently pull your leg toward your chest. Hold the stretch.
2. Change legs and repeat.

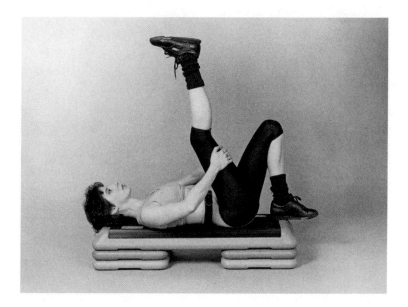

Chest Stretch

Lying on your back, bend your knees and place your feet close together on the bench or floor. Extend your arms out to the side slightly above shoulder level. With your hands palms up, reach down and back toward the floor. Hold the stretch.

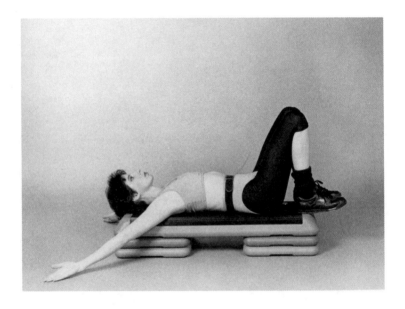

Back Stretch

Lying on your back, hug your knees into your chest. Hold
the stretch.

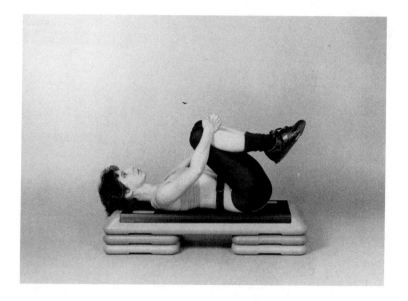

Quadriceps Stretch

1. Lying on your stomach, bring your right heel toward your right buttock. Simultaneously place your right hand on the instep of your right foot and press the instep into your hand. Hold the stretch.
2. Change legs and repeat.

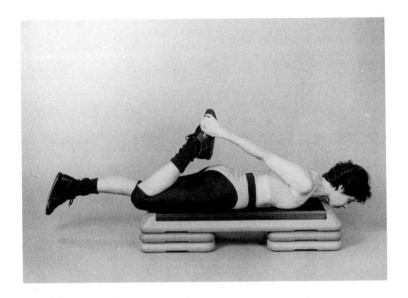

Shoulder Stretch

1. Sitting on the bench with both feet flat on floor, hold your right wrist with your left hand and pull your right arm across your chest. Hold the stretch.
2. Change arms and repeat.

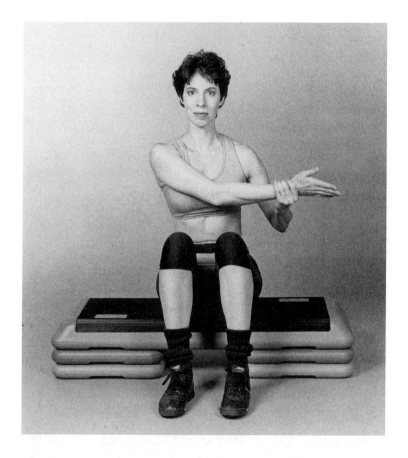

Triceps Stretch

1. Sitting on the bench with your feet flat on the floor, bend both arms over your head. Place your right hand on the upper back between your shoulder blades. Use your left hand to pull the right elbow gently toward the head. Hold the stretch.
2. Change arms and repeat.

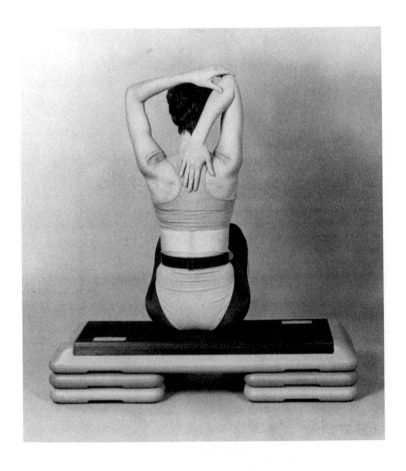

8

THE STEP TEST FOR
AEROBIC FITNESS

T o test your current level of cardiorespiratory fitness and monitor how the Bench Workout is improving your aerobic endurance, take a step test. This three-minute test, developed by Dr. Fred Kasch of San Diego, uses a postexercise heart rate or recovery heart rate as an indicator of fitness. The more fit you are, the faster your heart rate returns to normal.

Here's what you'll need for the test:

- A twelve-inch bench
- A watch with a second hand or a stopwatch
- A metronome (optional but useful for pacing your steps)

You should be rested before taking the step test. This means that any exercise that elevates your heart rate *should not* be done prior to the test.

The step action for the test is quite easy—step up with your right foot, step up with your left foot, step back down with the right foot, step back down with the left foot. This represents one full cycle. Practice the cycle a couple of times to acquaint yourself with the pattern.

The pacing of the steps is ninety-six beats per minute

(here's where the metronome is handy), which translates into twenty-four step cycles per minute. You may want to ask a friend to clap out the beats to help you keep your pace steady.

Once you're ready to begin . . .

1. Set a timer for three minutes and start the test.
2. Immediately after three minutes, sit down on the bench. NOTE: If at any time during the test you feel dizzy or light-headed or begin gasping for breath, stop the test immediately.
3. Within five seconds of sitting down, count your heart rate for one minute by monitoring your pulse at the radial (wrist) or carotid (neck) artery.
4. Use the recovery heart rate chart that follows to see how you score.

ONE-MINUTE RECOVERY HEART RATE
THREE-MINUTE STEP TEST

Rating	Men*	Women*
Excellent	90 or less	84 or less
Good	99–102	90–97
Above average	103–112	106–109
Average	120–121	118–119
Below average	123–125	122–124
Fair	127–130	129–134
Poor	136–138	137–145

*For ages 20–46.

Source: Adapted from *Y's Way to Physical Fitness,* Chicago: The YMCA of USA, 1982. Reprinted with permission from the YMCA of the USA, 101 North Wacker Drive, Chicago, IL 60606.

Congratulations on completing the Bench Workout! You've done a super job conditioning your body.

The workout, with its health benefits, body-shaping effects, and energy boost, offers a motivation to stay committed to exercise. Remember that you can use the Bench Workout to satisfy the weekly fitness guidelines for cardiovascular conditioning or combine it in a cross-training regimen of several different activities.

Most important, however, is that you have fun while you exercise—that's an essential part of any fitness program. With some upbeat music, challenging routines, and your own enthusiasm, you can make every workout a dynamic experience.

Keep up the good work and stay fit and healthy!